GRACEFUL AGING

LIVING YOUR OLD AGE TO THE FULLEST!

AUTHOR: DR. AIMEE JOSH MCDONALD

Table of Contents

INTRODUCTION

What Gentle Aging Entail

There are always at least a few magazine articles about how to look younger when you are in the checkout line. There's so much more to aging healthily, even though some wrinkles and sagging are what most people fear.

Living your best life and being in good enough physical and mental health to appreciate it are the keys to aging gracefully, not attempting to look like a twenty something. With proper maintenance, you can age better than a bottle of wine.

Continue reading to learn what to do and what not to do in your endeavor to age gracefully.

PART ONE

How to age gracefully

You may age gracefully from the inside out by using these strategies.

1. Treat your skin with kindness

Your body's largest organ is your skin. It may better shield your body from the weather, control body temperature, and provide feeling if you take good care of it.

To maintain optimal appearance and functionality:

1. When you're outside, put on protective clothes and sunscreen.

2. Get screened for skin cancer every year.

3. When it comes to your anti-aging skin care regimen, stick to moderate products.

4. Remain Hydrated

2. Workout

Frequent exercise helps you maintain your mobility for a longer period of time and dramatically reduces your risk of diseases like cancer and heart disease. In addition, exercise enhances mood, skin and bone health, sleep quality, and reduces stress.

Adults are advised by the Department of Health and Human Services to:

1.25 to 2.5 hours of vigorous-intensity aerobic activity per week, 2.5 to 5 hours of moderate-intensity exercise per week, or a combination of the two muscle-strengthening activities of moderate effort or higher, including all major muscle groups, twice a week or more, are recommended.

Here are a few instances of aerobic exercise:

- Strolling

- Swimming
- Dancing
- Cyclizing

Resistance bands or weights can be used for activities that strengthen bones and muscles.

In addition to cardiovascular and muscle-strengthening workouts, older persons should prioritize balance-training activities.

3. Pay attention to your diet

Eating a healthy diet is the key to ageing gracefully. According to the Dietary Guidelines for Americans, you should eat: vegetables and fruits, canned, frozen, or otherwise.

Lean protein—fish and beans, for example—at least three ounces of whole-grain breads, cereals, rice, or pasta each day, along with three servings of dairy products that are either fat-free or low-fat and fortified with vitamin D.

Good fats
For cooking, utilize oils rather than solid fats. Avoid refined sweets, processed meals, and harmful fats.

Reduce your intake of salt as well if you want to lower your blood pressure.

4. Mental wellness is important.

Living a joyful and stress-free life contributes significantly to aging well.

To maintain a positive attitude:

Spend time with your loved ones and friends. Strong social networks and meaningful interactions enhance longevity and promote both physical and mental health. Remember your furry family members; studies have shown that owning a pet lowers blood pressure and stress levels as well as reduces loneliness and improves mood.

Recognize your age. Research suggests that those with a positive outlook on aging have longer lifespans and may heal from disabilities more effectively. Understanding that aging is inevitable can have a profound impact.

Engage in activities you find enjoyable. Spending time doing things you enjoy can only increase your level of happiness. Whatever makes you happy, do it: take up a new activity, volunteer, or spend time in nature.

5. Continue to exercise

A sedentary lifestyle has been associated in numerous studies with a higher risk of chronic illness and premature death.

Taking vacations, joining group exercise programs, and going on walks and treks are a few ways to keep active.

6. Reduce your anxiety

Stress has a wide range of negative impacts on your body, from wrinkles and early aging to an increased chance of heart disease.

Many tried-and-true methods exist for reducing stress, such as:

+ Using methods of relaxation including yoga, breathing exercises, and meditation

+ Working Out

+ Getting enough rest

+ Conversing with a friend

7. Give up smoking and cut back on booze

It has been demonstrated that drinking alcohol and smoking both accelerate aging and raise the risk of disease.

Although giving up smoking is difficult, there are tools available to support you in your efforts. Consult a physician for advice on quitting.

Regarding alcohol, keep your use within the suggested range to prevent health hazards. That equates to one drink for women and two for men each day.

8. Get adequate rest

You need quality sleep for both your physical and emotional well-being. It affects the condition of your skin as well.

Your age determines the amount of sleep you require. Aim for seven to eight hours of sleep each night if you're an adult over the age of 18.

Sleeping sufficiently has been demonstrated to:

- Reduce the chance of stroke and heart disease

- Diminish anxiety and melancholy

- Reduce the likelihood of obesity

- Diminish inflammatory response

- Boost your ability to concentrate and focus.

9. Discover new interests

Throughout your life, discovering new and fulfilling interests can help you stay engaged and have a feeling of purpose.

Research indicates that those who participate in hobbies, leisure activities, and social gatherings live longer, are happier, and have less depression.

Maintaining a sense of purpose might be aided by taking up significant new interests.

10. Incorporate mindfulness

Acceptance and present-focused living are key components of mindfulness. Being aware offers several scientifically supported health advantages that can improve your aging process, such as:

- Enhanced concentration

- Improved recall

- Reduced tension

- Enhanced capacity for emotional response

- Relationship contentment

- Enhanced immunological response

Try these to cultivate mindfulness:

+ Meditating

+ Yoga

+ Chi tai

+ Painting

+ Reading

11. Sip lots of water

Getting adequate water enhances your energy and cognitive performance, as well as helping you stay regular. It has also been demonstrated to improve skin health and lessen aging symptoms.

Your recommended water intake is based on:

- You're thirsty

- Your degree of activity

- How frequently you move your bowels and urinate

- How much perspiration do you have?

- Which gender are you?

If you are unsure or worried about how much water you are consuming, consult a physician.

12. Look for your oral health

In addition to making your smile look older, not taking proper care of your teeth increases your risk of developing gum disease, which has been connected to bacterial pneumonia, heart attacks, and strokes.

Regular dental visits are essential in addition to good oral hygiene.

A dentist can identify symptoms of infections, cancer, malnutrition, and other disorders like diabetes, according to the American Dental Association. They advise using a mouth rinse, brushing twice a day, and flossing once a day.

13. Consult a physician frequently

Regular medical checkups can assist the physician in identifying issues early on or even before they arise. Your age, way of life, medical history, and current ailments all influence how frequently you visit the doctor.

As you get older, find out from your doctor how frequently you should get checks and screenings. Additionally, consult a physician whenever you have unsettling symptoms.

PART TWO

Where to look for assistance

Even though growing older is a natural part of life, some people find it challenging to adapt to these changes.

It's critical to get help if you're experiencing health concerns, finding it difficult to embrace aging, or fear that you're not aging gracefully.

Speak with a trusted person, like a member of your family or a close friend. You can also get professional assistance from a physician or counselor.

CONCLUSION

Being happy and healthy is more important for graceful aging than avoiding wrinkles.

Keep up a healthy lifestyle, spend time with the people you care about, and engage in activities that make you happy.

It's normal to be concerned about the difficulties that aging may present, so don't be afraid to voice your worries to someone.